Twelve Spoons

Riley Boerger

Enhanced DNA Publishing

DenolaBurton@EnhancedDNA1.com

www.enhanceddnapublishing.com 317-537-1438

Twelve Spoons

Editor: Katherine Walsh

Library of Congress Control Number: 2022945113

ISBN: 978-1-7378090-0-5

This book is based on real events. Names have been changed to protect the privacy of those in this story.

contents

DEDICATION AND THANK YOUS

In my fifteen years of life, I have met and been helped by so many people. Here are the ones who helped me the most:

Mrs. Lambert (My 8th-grade Challenge English and History Teacher): After years of being told I would never be a good writer, you were the first teacher and mentor to believe in what I wanted to say and that it had meaning. I will never be able to tell you how grateful I am for you in my life.

Mr. Fraser (My 9th-grade Speech and Debate Teacher): You made me believe I had a story that needed to be told, and that I could be proud of my differences. So, thank you, for always being there to talk to me and always giving me a platform to speak.

Madison (My Sister): You always supported me while also bringing me back down to Earth. I love you so much!

John Green (The author of my personal 'An Imperial Affliction') : Because pain demands to be felt.

Natalia (My best friend): We have been through hell together, but I will never forget the look on your face when I told you I was going to be a published author. Thank you for always pushing me further. I love you so much!

Enhanced Publishing DNA (Specifically Denola): Thank you for giving me a chance to make a dream come true.

Mom (My Hero): When people ask me who gave me the strength to fight every day without giving up, I always say, "My mom." Thank you for everything you have given me and supported me through. I love you to the moon and back.

And of course, to everyone else who made me who I am today, thank you. And thank you to my illness, because I won't have a book without it.

ACKNOWLEDGMENTS

This story is based on true events that happened to the author, but the personal details have been changed for readers' viewing.

I wrote this book for anyone who has ever been told their physical symptoms are all in their head.

I wrote this book for the people who know what the low FODMAP diet is.

I wrote this book for the early morning doctors' appointments, patients, and the teens who are rethinking their future because of their health.

I wrote this book for people going to appointments alone. The people who have never cried in the hospital, but the car is a different scenario.

I wrote this book for everyone out there who has lost friends and members of their families because they "didn't know how hard it would be to be in your life."

For the morning/night pill takers, and the people who know their physical therapy exercises like the back of their hand.

I wrote this book so we, as chronic pain/illness warriors, have a book to relate to. Because when I started to decline, I turned toward cancer books, and I would highlight them and annotate, but it always felt weird to relate to someone dying when I am not. This book is for everyone to annotate and highlight, to relate and share. I wrote this book because we don't have to be alone; we don't have to suffer in silence. I wrote this book because I'm a chronic pain/illness warrior.

present day

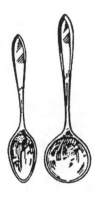

The truth is you never know what it's like to lose an ability you never knew you had. For me, it was the ability to walk pain-free.

As I walked into Seattle Children's Northern Clinic, my mask filled with the smell of hand sanitizer and rubbing alcohol. I shift my backpack just slightly and pull my ponytail just a little bit tighter.

"Ruth Bilbruck, 7/27/2007," I said, as I reached the front desk.

"I know who you are, Ruth," said Chase as he checked me over the hospital database. "I'm guessing there are no changes."

"Nope."

After coming here three times a week for six months, I think they should know I don't have measles or chickenpox.

"K, here's your wristband, you know the rest," Chase said, handing me a purple wristband with my patient information on it.

I head to the waiting area and sit down. In the waiting room at Seattle Children's Northern Clinic, there are three undefined sections. In the front near the windows are the toddlers and babies with their parents. The middle section is for children to teens who come in with their parents. And the back section is for the teens who have been sick for so long that they come to treatments by themselves, and that's where I sit.

I pull out my earbuds and start some music to distract myself from what is soon to happen. Next to the waiting area is the Physical Therapy gym, which I know all too well. Behind that is the Biofeedback room, where I used to do my treatment before I was released from that program. The sharp stabbing pain radiates down my legs as I adjust my position. I sit there quietly for what feels like thirteen years, thinking about what I have been through these past years. The needles, exercises, tests, and treatments. The people I have met and the bonds I have created, most having to leave to move on to new treatments.

Never knowing that I had to leave till the day I did. Every six weeks I have to go to my doctor, though the pain continued...

"Ruth, Ruth, RUTH!" a voice said. They have been trying to get my attention for a long time, I guess.

"Hmm, Oh, hey." Turning, I see my physical therapist of six months looking minimally impressed with my keen hearing. "Mark, hey."

Mark looked at me and motioned toward the hall. I collect my things and start to move toward the opening. As I walk into the Physical Therapy Gym, my eyes fall onto the blue and orange accents that highlight the different walls. Treatment tables surround the border of the open concept room, and in the middle sits an elliptical, treadmill, and stationary bike. At the side of the room sits a large workout mat with a large mirror in front of it, and there is a bathroom down the hallway toward the therapist's office. I feel this wave of dread wash over me. The same feeling I had when I entered this room for the first time almost six months ago. As I set down my Stranger Things Loungefly bag and my emotional support water bottle, Mark asks me which machine I would like to start my workout on. I respond with, "None, I want to take a nap."

Which apparently was the wrong answer. He chose the treadmill. I step onto the machine I have walked over twenty miles on easy mode. I settle into my normal pattern: step on the machine, clip in, grab sidebars, and wait for Mark to choose what setting I am on today. Today he chose hills, which made me shoot him an 'if looks could kill you would be dead' glare. It's the setting he usually chooses, but for some reason, it still surprises me. As I start to walk, I look out the large floor-length window in front of me.

It's a beautiful summer day, and I appreciate the picture-perfect sunrise as it's a nice break from the blank gym walls.

"What have you been up to recently?" Mark asks while charting my speed and settings. My legs already grow tired, which is not a good thing when I am only five minutes into my workout. That's the way it has been recently. My legs feel weaker every day, and the pain continues to spread. I wake up and my body is already fighting itself, having fire pains spread through my whole body. Somedays, it's so bad I curl up in a ball and stay in bed. Most days, it's the first of many battles I face.

"School, mostly," I respond, turning my attention back to my walking as I started to get a little wobbly. Who knew it took so much concentration to walk on something as simple as a moving platform? "Trig is kicking my butt. Why do I have to know *tan*, *cos*, and *sin*? How many times a day do you use the unit circle to solve a problem?" I asked.

As I finish my rant, I let out a long breath. I try to hide it as a flustered exhale, but truthfully, I am kind of out of breath.

"I can tell you with 100 percent certainty that one, I have no idea what you are talking about. Which, in turn, means two, I probably won't ever use it," Mark responded, always joking around when he knows I am getting stressed.

Mark once told me every aspect of my life brings me stress, from my health, to school, to my home life. So, when I walk through those gym doors, I have to allow myself one hour of not worrying; one hour of carefree wonder; one hour to just be, not worrying about what my next steps are.

"Well, I guess that's good because after this year I am emptying my brain of all school," I responded, noticing the treadmill reads eight minutes. "I'm done," I said, jumping off the treadmill, almost forgetting to unclip. I walk over to pick up my water bottle, unscrewing the cap.

"What is engraved on your water bottle?" Mark asked, moving his desk over to the dashed floor.

"Ohh, it says 'Emotional Support Water Bottle'. It's a joke in my family because I take my water bottle everywhere with me, that's my emotional support water bottle. My aunt and uncle found it really funny and got this one custom-made for me," I said, showing him my forest green Yeti water bottle. "And the stickers are added by yours truly." I said, pointing to my favorite one, a depiction of Loki from the Marvel universe with words around him saying, "I have been falling for thirty minutes."

As I walk over to meet Mark, I realize what is about to happen.

"What do you want to start off with, maybe bear walks?" Mark said with a mischievous smile.

I rolled my eyes at him but assumed the bear walk pose: hands and feet on the floor, walk out with my hands, then inch worm my feet until they met my hands, and then do it all over again. I once counted. It was about twenty times down and twenty times back.

This is my least favorite workout.

As I finish it, I stand up and look at Mark, "I hate you," I said, twisting to stretch out my back.

"You'll like me someday in the future. Maybe while you're walking down the aisle at your wedding and you don't have to stop halfway through because your back is not hurting." Mark said, listing off my next exercise.

After I finish my warm-up, Mark tells me to get on the elliptical. "What is the number the speed needs to be over?" Mark asks.

"Sixty-five," I mumbled, remembering the first time he t _____ that number.

"And what happens if it goes below that number for more than three seconds?"

"The timer starts over," I said, turning on the machine.

It takes me a minute to get into the normal phase, but once I do, eight minutes go by in a flash. The elliptical is my least favorite of the machines we work on, but it's manageable. I grab my water again and take a long sip. Screwing on the lid, I ask Mark, "What's next?" He shows me some new at-home workouts: child pose, bird dog, hamstring stretch. And then our forty-five minutes are up. I run to the bathroom to get changed; I am expected at school shortly after leaving the gym.

When I enter the bathroom, I walk over and set my bag on the table. I look at myself in the mirror. There are dark crescent moons under my eyes, hair that is very due for a wash, and my neck and arms are corpse pale. All reminders that I am a person living with a chronic illness. I look like a Skrull from Captain Marvel. My cheeks are less full than they were a year ago. I pull out my green crew neck sweatshirt and my pair of black leggings. After getting changed, I pull my short, brown hair into a high ponytail and place my necklace and black moon earrings at their prospective places. I pull a couple strands of hair loose from the tight rubber band to frame my face as best as I can. I splash my face with water, trying to wake myself up as it is 7:40 a.m. I have been up since 5:45 a.m. I pull out my little makeup bag I keep in my hospital bag, a benign tote with a patch on it, and I reapply my eyeliner and mascara. I stare in the mirror and say to myself, "It's not great, but it's not horrible." Once I am done I scan the room, making sure I have not forgotten anything, and I make my way out of the bathroom, closing the door behind me.

"I'm out," I said, waving at Mark. "I'll see you on Thursday!"

"Yep, have a good day at school!" Mark said, while wiping down a table for the next patient.

As I exit the gym, I wave at my Biofeedback Specialist, George, and make my way to the waiting room. I look for Chase; we usually talk before I leave. I see he is busy with another patient, so instead, I wave and leave the building.

two years prior

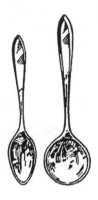

As my mom parks, she grabs my hand. "Are you sure you don't want me to come in with you?"

"No Mom, I'll be fine really, and if you need proof, you can watch me through the wall of windows facing the parking lot," I said, sarcastically pointing over my shoulder to the building behind me. It is one of the buildings in a little strip mall. I have been here before. My favorite trampoline park is just down the way.

"You'll just be sitting there, in the corner, bored and uncomfortable. Stay here in the AC and comfortable seats." I said, reaching over to kiss my mom.

As the baby of the family, she has been, and probably will always be, very protective of me. Especially when it comes to anything related to my health. I grab my blue water bottle out of the drink holder and open the door.

"I love you, Mom."

"I love you, too, honey." My mom said, while signing, I love you in American Sign Language.

Since I was three years old, whenever my mom dropped me off or I went somewhere, we would voice and sign to each other, "I love you." It was her way of not being that parent screaming, "I LOVE YOU" at her children as she's driving away. Even though there were a couple of situations where that happened. As I pull open the heavy door to the new PT gym, I look around, truly unimpressed with how it looked. I mean, it looked like every other physical therapy place I have ever been to. Practical Physical Therapy was the new physical therapy gym Doctor Pollen transferred me to after our first visit. It's been a little over a month since my hip started to hurt, and this is already the second physical therapist I have seen. I am getting impatient, hoping that I will receive answers soon.

I am greeted by an older, blonde woman at the front desk. "Hi, how can I help you today?" She asked, smiling

"Hi, I'm Ruth Bilbruck. I'm here to see Diana House," I replied, saying the last name a little louder than the rest.

I'm a longtime Dr. House fan. The fact that my new physical therapist was a Doctor of Physical Therapy, meaning legally she was Dr. House, made me fangirl just a little bit.

"Sounds good, and it's your first time here, correct?" She said, reaching behind her to grab an actual paper file with my name on it.

Where in the twenty-first century do people still use paper files? Isn't everything digital?

"Yes."

"Well, because of that, we have some paperwork. A Physical therapist will come and get you warmed up, and then Diana will see you," she said, passing me a clipboard with the papers and a pen with their logo.

"Thanks," I said, grabbing the clipboard and pen, then taking a seat.

Physical therapy paperwork is so boring and it's always the same things. When did the pain start? How old are you? Where is the pain? Sign here to approve the kidnapping of your first child. Always the same. I chuckle to myself, reminding myself to tell my best friend that joke later. Right as I finish the last piece of paper, a thin man comes over and calls my name. "Hi, that's me," I said, standing and grabbing my water bottle. I hand the man the clipboard as he introduces himself.

"Hi, my name is Roger. I am one of the two assistant PTs that work here, and I'm going to get you warmed up."

"Hi, I'm Ruth. As you know from the paperwork, and that sounds fantastic, thank you." I responded, as we pulled up near a stationary bike.

As I sit down, Roger goes over my medical history hoping nothing has changed. To his luck, nothing has. I have never had a surgery or a long-term health issue. I am on no medication or therapies they need to know of. I'm a normal kid with some hip pain that will be resolved soon. I finish up on the bike, Roger points to a table and tells me to put my stuff on it. I do as I am told and drop off my water bottle and phone. There is a low possibility that I will need either of them in the next forty minutes.

"K, you are all set. I will tell Diana that you are warmed up and ready to meet with her. And then once you are done with that, I will be back to explain and supervise the workouts she assigned to you." Roger said, while wiping down the table next to me with disinfectant.

"Sounds great, thank you."

It only took a couple minutes before a taller woman with dark brown hair pulled into a low ponytail is heading my way. She pulls up a swivel stool and opens her laptop, which I assume is where she keeps her patient notes.

"Are you Ruth Bilbruck?" She asked, reaching out her hand for a handshake.

"Yeah," I said, shaking it back. "It's very nice to meet you."

"You as well. So, tell me a little bit about what is going on that brought you here today," she said, typing down something really quick.

"Well, about a month ago, I started getting really sharp hip pain in my right hip. This followed trying to correct my walk per my doctor's request."

"Ok, and what were they trying to fix?" She asked, continuing to type, but somehow still looking at me.

"I walk with my feet pointed outwards, like a duck, and I have since I was a child, but my doctor thought it would be valuable to correct the way I walk as it would prevent further damage in the future," I explain, rubbing my arm up and down, as it is my anxiety response.

"When did they start trying to correct it?"

"When I was nine."

"Seriously?" Diana said surprised, "At that age, your hip joints are basically completely secure and reinforced, the only way to fix your walk at that age would be to break your hip joint, then realign the joint, and then go through physical therapy to correct it. But for someone who is not having any problems walking now, I would never recommend that course of treatment for a person."

"Well, my doctor did. And when I was trying, my hip started to hurt, and once I stopped, it continues to hurt." I said, slowing down the rubbing of my arm.

"Well, if you don't mind, I would like to start with using cupping to try to stretch out the muscles around the joint. Then you and Roger are going to work on strengthening and stretching out your back and hip. Sounds good?"

I nodded, lying down on my left side. When she comes back, she has these suction devices, towels, and shea butter. She places towels in the elastic of my shorts and the hem of my shirt, pulling them in opposite ways. She applies some of the shea butter.

As she does, I feel transported back to being a 7-year-old going to physical therapy for plantar fasciitis pain. The PT used it to massage out the arch and ball of my feet. It's one of those smells I correlate with my childhood, but I have never been able to pinpoint the source, until now.

Diana places the first cupping tool on my hip, my back slightly arches in pain.

"Is that ok?" Diana asked, pulling it off.

"Yeah, it's fine, sorry," I replied, lowering my body back onto the table.

As she moves the tool, I feel my nerves firing all over my body, not just in my hip. That's not normal. I ball my left hand into a fist and grab my left hand with my right hand. Doing so leaves nail indents after she finishes.

"We're done!" Diana said, removing the towels and throwing them into a basket behind her.

"K, thanks!" I replied, sitting up slowly.

I can already tell my back will be pretty tight. When I fully sit up and twist my back, I can feel the popping travel down my spine. *Wow, that felt really good.* Diana walks over to the printer and returns with a stapled packet of what I assume are my new physical therapy exercises. I reach out for the paper and grab it, flipping through the pages. *Man, why couldn't they just be stretches?*

"So, I want you to do the stretches twice a day and then the strengthening exercises once a day. And I want your return to gym visits to be twice a week, for six weeks. Then we will reevaluate." Diana said, grabbing a business card to hand to me. "If you have any questions, please don't hesitate to call. It was very nice meeting you today, and I will see you next week."

I reach out my hand to shake, "Thank you, yeah I will."

As Roger comes over, I stand and shake out my hands like I have done a million times. *Man, it is too early, and I am under-caffeinated for this.*

present day

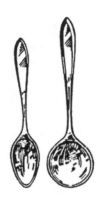

I grab the red clip and place it on my bra strap through my shirt. Clipping in means that if I pass out or fall, the machine will immediately stop, and I am not left with a beautiful treadmill mark.

"Why do I have to clip in?" I ask Mark, "I already have beautiful tread marks from when I was younger, and my friends and I played on her treadmill. She poured marbles on it while I was running at level ten," I said turning my chin up to show him the dent that was taken out of my chin years earlier.

"I'm not going to answer that," Mark answers, turning the treadmill to hills and then stepping back and writing something on his laptop.

"What are you writing? A note to Dr. Bloom asking to have a discussion about my excessive need to question everything we do here?"

Dr. Bloom is my pain psychologist. The best way to describe him is a mix between Dr. House from *House, M.D.* and Dr. Cox from *Scrubs*.

"Haha, will you please concentrate on your walking? I made you wear the clip, but that doesn't mean I want you to have to use it." Mark responds while placing his hand on my lower back to adjust how I am walking.

I continue to walk for about a minute, concentrating on placing one foot in front of the other, just like a baby learning to walk.

"How is your work going with Dr. Wilson, by the way?" Mark asks, breaking the comfortable silence.

"Fine," I respond, continuing to concentrate on my feet.

One, Two, One,

Two, Left, Right, Left, Right.

My work with Dr. Wilson is weird. It's all breathing techniques and trying not to concentrate on the pain when I am having a flare-up. Which is like telling a soon-to-be mother in labor to not think of the child she will be pushing out of her vagina shortly.

"That's it?" Mark asks flabbergasted, "You can talk for an hour about Dr. House or *Grey's Anatomy*. But I ask you about YOUR medical treatment and you act like you have never spoken more than three words." I turn to look at him now, losing count of which foot I am on.

"What do you want me to say?" I ask, "Nothing is happening, and my pain is not getting any better, and for some reason, I continue to have hope every time I enter this facility. That it's been over two years since I started having pain, and now it's full body and my stomach hurts all the time, and I can't stop thinking about when it will end to start living again."

I take a long breath, not looking at Mark because I already know what he looks like. His eyes will have a pity fog over them, and his normal perfect posture will be replaced with a hunched-over stance because people think it makes them look more comforting.

"Ruth, I'm sorry. I didn't know that you were still struggling with that. Have you thought at all about seeing that therapist we talked about? I think it could be really helpful." Mark said, smiling.

Or I think he is smiling, but he's wearing a mask. He could be sticking his tongue out at me, and I would not know. I continue to walk.

"I don't need a shrink."

"Not a shrink, a therapist. Someone you could talk to about all of this, and might even be able to get you on some antidepressants?" Mark said.

"Nah, I'll pass. I'm too busy for one anyway," I replied.

One, Two, One, Two, Left, Right, left, Righ...

When I come to, I am on my back. My legs have been lifted above me on an elevation cube, and I have a cold washcloth on my forehead. My eyes start to focus. I see Mark kneeling over me.

"What happened?" I ask, trying to sit up.

My back seizes up. It's too painful to bend. I slowly lower myself back down to the ground.

"Hi, Ruth," a person I have never met before says. "Can you tell me your date of birth, please?"

"07/27/2007," I responded, confused. I turn to Mark. "What happened?"

"You passed out. You didn't get injured, but that's only because you were wearing the clip." He said, pointing to the red clip still attached to my sports bra. "Ruth, has this been happening?"

I'm slow to respond. Not because I hit my head, but because this was so *déjà vu*-ish, and because there were so many new people around. I was trying to process it all.

"Sorta, but mostly dizziness, not full passing out. I'll be fine." I replied, standing up and making my way to one of the PT tables.

My back usually hurts but falling down and having to lie on the floor did not aid it in any way. I lie there until the crowd of people disperses and it is just me and Mark. He is holding one of my arms to take my pulse. I sit up, trying to locate my water. My mouth is so dry I think *Aladdin* is being filmed in it.

"Where are you trying to go?" Mark asks.

"I want my water," I said, bending until I am up on my forearms. Mark brings it to me. "Thank you," I responded as he handed it to me. I twist the cap off and take a large swig. I can feel the large gulp flowing down my throat and into my stomach.

"Anything sore?" He asks, palpating my back.

"No, I'm good..," I respond, unintentionally wincing as he places his hand on my lower back.

"Liar," Mark said, pulling my shirt up to inspect the troubled area. "Wooo, that is going to leave a mark."

"Why is it always me, Mark? Why is it always me with health issues?" I asked, tearing up. "It feels like since the age of six I was always the medical child, and this illness just makes it worse."

"It's going to get better, Ruth. Just think, in a few months you are going to be laughing at this moment with your friends, pain-free."

one-and-a-half years prior

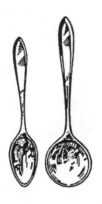

I'm sure it's not the healthiest thing I could be doing, but recently I have been spending a lot of time researching chronic pain. The information comes from hospital websites, personal blogs, and chat rooms. Stories of people accepting that they will live with chronic pain forever make the last shred of hope in me deflate like an untied balloon. I learned that when you live with chronic pain, you become a chronic illness warrior, and I like that. It does feel like every day I am fighting a dragon to stay alive. The dragon is my own body. My weapons are medications, regimens, and medical appointments.

I also found this theory called the Spoon Theory, originally created by Christine Miserandino, as a way to explain what it was like living with Lupus. Now it is used across the chronic illness community. The theory is that people with chronic illness start the day with twelve spoons. Everything costs a spoon. So, getting up in the morning is one spoon, exercising is worth three spoons, etc. This theory visualizes the need to conserve energy, or spoons, if you are living with a chronic illness. The number of spoons you start the day with changes. If you didn't sleep well the night before, you start off with six spoons. If your medication is not working well, maybe you have only three spoons. Now the first time I heard it, I didn't like it. I couldn't believe that people were living their lives based off cutlery. Right now, as the pain has gotten worse, I completely get it. I notice since reading the article; I have been using it a lot more. If my friends invite me to hang out after school but I have homework, I calculate how many spoons it will take up. Hanging out with friends will cost me four spoons, homework is three, and I could do both, but that would mean I wouldn't sleep well tonight. So, I think it will be better for me to stay home and do my homework, so I have my twelve spoons tomorrow. This theory also makes it easier to explain it to my friends and family. No one truly understands what this is like, other than people going through it themselves — fellow spoonies.

PResenT Day

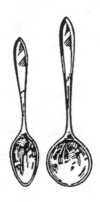

As I get into the car, I turn and look at my mom.

"How was Mark?" my mother asks, removing her purse from my place in the shotgun seat.

"He's good, more sarcastic than ever, but good," I said, placing my water bottle and purse between my legs.

I complain about Mark, but truly, he is one of the reasons I am still alive today. About a year ago, I was in a really dark place. He told me to call the number on his card if I needed anything because I deserve the right to grow up and live an amazing life.

So, though I complain, I could never thank him enough, though I would never tell him that.

I lie my head against the car headrest and take my first full breath of the day. I click on my phone to see a text from my best friend, Nellie.

Hey girl, how was physical therapy? How's Mark, any fun Mark Story's? Also, do you want to come over tonight and watch the new Grey's episode? Let me know! Love you!

Nellie always knows the right thing to say, I think. After physical therapy and being on this new medication, I don't think I would be up for it. All I want right now is a cup of coffee and a good book.

Hey love, Physical therapy was good! I'm saving the Mark stories for the next time we see each other! Thanks for the invitation but I just finished physical therapy and these nerve blockers are kicking my ass, another time though! Love!

I click off my phone and place it back into my bag.

"Are you ok? You look really pale," my mom asks while pulling out of the parking lot.

"Yeah, I'm fine," I respond, taking a sip of water. "Probably just dehydrated. Do you have any clients today?"

My mom owns her own interior design business, which is really helpful. She can kind of make her own schedule, but that does mean she is the only one with TONS of clients.

"No, I have to work on the Pattel project though," my mom said, trying to not have the boredom be heard in her voice.

"Nice, well your day sounds busy," I replied, opening Instagram.

My phone is instantly filled with account after account of people living their best lives. Pictures of kids my age at parties and with their significant other make me feel sicker than when I forget to take my anti-nausea meds. That's one of the reasons I don't like social media. I know that makes me sound old, but I have real-life 'fear of missing out'. I know I'm missing normal teenage experiences. Social media just makes it worse. That's why I kind of use my platforms as a reality check for all the people following me or come across my page. I use it as a 'look at me hanging off the side of my bed with no makeup on and clothes that I have not changed in two days kind of thing.' Because "normal" life is not always brunches and filtered photos. Especially my life. Living with a chronic illness is not glamorous. I open my story and take a quick photo of myself sitting in the car, then I write out a quick message.

Just finished Physical Therapy, I am SOOOO tired. All I want right now is a cup of coffee and the new @ColleenHoover book. #CHRONICALLYILLNESS #CHRONICALLYBADASS

I click the post button and then turn off my phone as my mother pulls into Starbucks.

"How do you always read my mind?" I ask her.

"What?" she said, turning toward me, grabbing her purse out of the backseats.

"I literally just posted on my Instagram story that all I want is coffee and the new Colleen Hoover book," I said pulling up the post to prove it.

"I don't know, I guess it's just my mother instinct," she said.

At home, I am attacked by my dog, Colleen, as I walk through the front door. In my family, we name our animals after authors. I got to choose Colleen's name, as you might have guessed. I head to my bedroom, the basement of the house. Colleen chases after me. She gallops into my room as I open the door, flinging herself onto my bed. Colleen is a Great Anatolian-Pyrenees mix, so she's huge. She has the sweetest face and eyeliner that every makeup wearer is jealous of. I put my bag on the hook it lives on, and collapse on my bed, wrapping myself in more blankets than I could count.

My room is best described as a collection of all things around me. I created my room when I started to get sick. I wanted a sanctuary of things I love. I spend more time in it than in any other place in the world. On the back of my door hangs a collage of over fifty *Grey's Anatomy* pictures; on the wall next to that is a *New Girl* tapestry. On the same wall hangs my collection of cow pictures, all in different mediums. On either side of my windowsill houses my large collection of Funko Pops. A glass whiteboard hangs from the wall across from my bed next to my folding desk. Each aspect of my room was chosen and/or created by me. I believe that my room should be my happy place, my calm, as my life is the storm. I pull out one of my black silk sleep masks and turn on my fan. I try to get comfortable to take a nap. That is a ritual for me after physical therapy: come home, say hi to Colleen, and then nap time. As usual, my appointment was at 7:30 a.m. I choose to believe it was just a break in my sleep from the night before. My eyes start to grow heavy, and just like that, I am asleep.

My dreams have always been weird, but ever since I started taking all the meds, they have become even weirder. The most recurring dreams goes like this:

I wake up and I reach to take my morning medication; my pill organizer is gone. I get up and open my dresser where I keep my medical basket; it is gone. Around the room my foam roller, braces, walking boots, and TENS unit, are replaced by books, clothes, and makeup. I get out of my room, then I realize I'm not in any pain, my back feels good, and my stomach feels hungry, which hasn't happened in a long time. I make myself a breakfast full of my trigger foods, bacon, pancakes, and coffee. After eating like it was my first meal in forever, I realize I feel no GI pain, no nausea, and no acid reflux. I'm okay. I open my phone and see that my Tiktok handle Chronically_Ruth has been replaced with Iconically_Ruth. I post videos of myself dancing, not chronic illness awareness videos. I put on the running shoes that I used to wear every day. They are not collecting dust, and go for a run. I reach the two-mile mark. I sit down on top of a hill by my house and watch the sunrise. It's so beautiful; it's like the days of illness and pain were just a bad dream. I start to cry. I am so happy. I am so ok. I am so perfect.

Then I wake up, and it's obviously a dream. I remove my eye mask and I realize I have been crying. Which is the same thing that has happened the other hundreds of times I had that dream. I never realize how much I miss my old life. When you have a chronic illness, you are always told that you will mourn your own life. Just like mourning a person, that process is not linear.

I think I will be perfectly fine with my new normal someday. Other days, it feels like my life ended that day I saw my doctor.

Four Months Prior

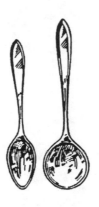

A couple months ago, I joined an online chronic illness support group per my therapist, Morgan's, recommendation. I was not for the idea, but Nellie brought up a good point. "You could find your Augustus Waters." So, I gave in and joined the Facebook group. Even though I have yet to find my Gus, it's been going great. I didn't understand how helpful it would be to have people who are going through what I am. Whenever I am stressed or having a flare-up, I can turn to them to be my second pair of ears. We use Facebook messenger to talk so it's not something where we have to wait to talk, it's constantly being used. Questions, comments, even personal wins are shared on it. Twenty-three of us use it daily, and we are from all over the world. I used to think it was cringy, or I was making a big deal out of my illness. It's something I suffer with; I have had to learn to deal with it. I no longer feel guilty. A normal chat goes a little something like this:

Tiana: Overworking myself for my music but still doing it bc I don't know when to quit lmao, we love trying to make career as a teen

Ruth: Bru me too. I'm so tired, but I have more French to do.

Ash: That's me with writing content for my FB page at 2 am

Tiana: It's addicting but also burns me out so much to keep posting music

Ruth: I think a lot of us are addicted to it because we feel like we need to be doing something with our lives. Sending love and spoons

Ash: People expect me to post often. So much pressure to write interesting and informative posts. Always burning out now

Ash: One side note, soon I'll reach 1000 followers!! Considering I only started it in April, that's pretty good

Tiana: That's really good!!! And yeah I get the burnt out part

Tiana: Gotta remember to take breaks but it's hard.

Abby: I'm super close to 4k but I use Instagram more, I'm not sure if you can do it here but you can "prewrite" posts and save them as drafts and it's such a huge help!!! If you're feeling good you can bang out a few to save for later

Emma: They have that on Facebook too

Abby: Definitely use it to your advantage then!

Ash: Yeah I do that... at 2 am

Tiana: Smarrttt, doesn't apply to be exactly for writing but I can make videos (a few in advance) and post them

To anyone on the outside, that might mean nothing. To all these amazing, strong, and inspiring people, it's a community that we all need in our lives. Most people can't fully understand what it is like to live a life full of pain or doctors' appointments. When we complain to them, they tell us they are sorry and that we will get better someday. But in this group, we understand that if someone is complaining, they just need to hear, 'We hear you and we will not try to fix what you are going through, but we are here for you to tell your struggles to'. This group of people is my lifeline. We never have enough time in a day to talk. They are the first text in the morning and the last text every night. My support and love. My spoonies and people. They are who I turn to for support, and I am forever thankful for them.

present Day

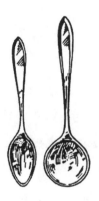

Today is my pain clinic evaluation and I already want to leave. It's five-ish hours of appointments, so I am missing school, but that's the only positive I can find. I sit in my hospital room at Seattle Children's Hospital. I start to notice the things on the walls; the reminders for parents to pick up their children's medications, or to ask the doctor about a note for school. They are obsolete to my mother and me. I have run on meds and hospital notes for years now, forgetting one would be like forgetting to breathe. I fidget with my purple hospital band, trying to memorize the patient ID number. Not because it is important or because it will improve my life in any way, just because I am bored. O*ne... five... six... two, ohh I give up*. I have had to wear over fifty of these purple hospital bands. Today, I can only remember my patient number starts with one. I open Google Classroom and my leadership Google Meet, hoping to catch the last ten minutes of work time. I also need to get my assignment from my leadership teacher, Mrs. Casey. But as usual, the internet at the hospital sucks. I can't load it, so I send her an email instead.

Dear Mrs. Casey,

As I reminded you yesterday I am at a full day doctor appointment today so I will be unable to be at class and/or attend the google meet. I know we are assigning jobs today so I was wondering if it would be possible for you to email me the project I will be working on and the name of the other students working on that project? Thank you so much, if you need anything today, feel free to email me. Have an amazing day.

Sincerely, Ruth Bilbruck

I press the send button and feel a wave of exhaustion come over me. *I am the only kid wishing they were at school today.* Even though I know this is for my health and will probably make it better, I still hate the idea that I will be here the whole day. I have so many things to do. Instead of freaking out, I pull out my daily planner and write a list.

- Wash Water Bottle

- Write paper for english

- Take Shower

- Send out welcome email to your project members

- Read chapters for history

- Send out senator meeting reminders

I close my book and turn when I hear two knocks at the door. Without even processing what is happening, I answer, "Come in."

An older gentleman and a younger woman walk in. The man's name is Dr. Wilson, the head director of Seattle Children's Pain Clinic. The woman's name is Dr. McMelson. They both pull up stools to ask the same fifteen questions I have been asked for the past two years. I shift slightly, preparing myself for the mind-numbing torture that was about to ensue. Chronic pain meetings are always the same questions:

1. How's the pain today on a scale from one to ten?

2. When did the pain start and when did it start to spread?

3. What treatments have you tried?

4. How do you deal with the pain?

5. What do you think causes it?

I'm like a robot answering the questions. Like an actor who has rehearsed their lines for years.

Of course, though there is always the 'I'm sorry' or 'Wow, you should not be having to go through this at such a young age.' Like I know, you think I'm doing this for the kicks and giggles? After we finish, Dr. Wilson throws in a new one. This question was not for me, it was for my mom.

"Mom, do you think you can explain your experience with Ruth's pain and what you think caused it?" Dr. Wilson asks.

I turn to my mom and notice that she is not preparing to speak. She is actually crying. I can't tell if it's because she is so happy we are finally at this appointment. She has been working so hard to get or if it's because my pain has really been affecting her so much. Either way, she was crying in the middle of the hospital after just one question. Dr. Wilson grabs the tissue box off the counter next to him and hands it to my mom. She accepts it. I start to feel bad. Aren't I supposed to be the one crying?

"Sorry," my mom said, dabbing her eyes with one of the tissues. "Her pain has not physically affected me, but every single day I am forced to watch my daughter live through constant pain, and I have to be strong for her, but it's really hard. And I'm not the one living with it, I'm just watching it happen. She needs some answers, we need some answers. I mean that's why we're here right, to help Ruth."

As she finishes, she turns to me and gives me a slight nod. Our way of telling each other 'I love you' without having to sign it.

"Yes, we are, and let's hope that after today we will have some answers for the both of you," Dr. McMelson replies, turning toward me. "I'm assuming the nurse gave you today's schedule?"

I nod.

"Great, so first you will meet with me, and I will do a full physical evaluation. And then you will meet with Dr. Wilson. And then you will head up to physical therapy to meet with our unit's physical therapist. Does that sound about right?"

"Sounds good."

"Great, well, we are both going to step out and I will be back in a minute. Do either of you have any questions?"

My mom and I shake our heads. The doctors leave. And so begins the longest day of my life.

SIX MONTHS PRIOR

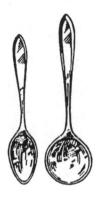

As my alarm rings, I turn over and grab my phone. The message I had titled the alarm with the night before blinds me it reads:

TODAY'S THE DAY, ENDOSCOPY DAY!!!

I still can't believe that I am fourteen and in less than three hours going to get an endoscopy. For those who do not know what that is, it's a surgical procedure where a long rope-like camera is threaded down your throat and into your upper intestines to check for lesions or ulcers. I have to get one because I have been having persistent, chronic GI pains for three months. They want to make sure it's not something acutely wrong. It's 4:45 a.m. and I need to check in at the Seattle Campus at 6:00 a.m. I need to leave in fifteen minutes. I grab the outfit I preplanned the night before and make my way to the bathroom. I wash my face, brush my teeth, put on deodorant, and get changed, and then I'm ready to go. I grab my pre-packed bag for the hospital off my chair and the 'in case I die cards' off my desk. As I walk upstairs, my knees start to shake out of anxiety. But I keep moving. I want to get the cards laid out before my mom comes downstairs. I choose a place that anyone will see, below the tv, and lay them out. One for my brother, sister-in-law, mom, sister, my four best friends, and my absent dad. I head to the entryway as I hear my mother walk down the stairs. "Morning," I said, checking my Instagram, and taking a fit check for my story.

"Morning, sweety!" My mom replied, hugging me. I can tell that she is scared. My mom hates all things medical. She watched both of her parents die in hospitals, so these things are not her favorite, but she does them for me.

"Mom, I can't breathe," I said, patting her back.

"Sorry, should we get going?"

"We shall," I said, opening the front door.

The car ride there was boring and oddly quiet. Usually, my mom and I used this time to talk and catch up. Today, we both had other things on our minds. I got to play my music, which is rare, so the car was filled with Bo Burnham, musical theater, and the random *Blackbear* song. We pull into the parking lot.

My mom reaches over to grab my hand. "We should pray." My mother is pretty religious. I am not. I know that this prayer is for her, not for me. I bow my head like I was taught from a young age, "Dear Heavenly Father, we pray today to ask you to watch over Ruth as she goes into this procedure today and to return her to us. We also pray for answers to come from this test, and we say this in your name, ah,"

"Men."

"Men."

I jump out of the car just in time, so my mom doesn't start prayer part two. The weather is cool for August. We walk down the stairs we have taken numerous times to get to the entrance. We are greeted by two women sitting with thermometers and the amazing 'screened for COVID stickers'. After we get checked, we have to get checked in. Once that's done, we are directed to go wait in the surgical waiting area. I sit down, trying to forget why I am here. I put in my earbuds and press play on my everyday playlist. "Memory" by *Blackbear* plays, and I lean my head against the seat and exhale. My mom is responding to text messages and scrolling through Facebook. Her way of dissociating, or escaping reality, just for a minute. I don't mind. If she asks me one more time how I am feeling, I'm going to kill her. My mother and I are one of two families there at this ungodly hour. I don't know why my mother thought this would be a good time to schedule this, but I also didn't ask. Her usual answer is, "I like to get them done early, and then you still have your whole day." I have never and will never agree with that. I'm more of a do your whole day then go to your doctor appt, so you get to go home and sleep. My mom drives me, so she gets to choose. The hospital is usually very bright and cheering. Now it is dark. It reminds me of movies where the couple has dinner under the candlelight. It's also quiet. I am used to the hospital being loud and bustling. It is anything but that. I can literally hear a pen drop. I feel a yawn creep up and let it out. My mom must have seen me because she reaches over and rubs my knee.

"Just think, in a matter of an hour, you will get the best sleep you have had in a long time."

"Yeah, I mean you're not wrong," I replied

"Ruth. Ruth" A woman I'm assuming is a nurse calls.

"That's me!" I said, standing up and walking to her. She reaches out to check my wristband, looking to confirm my patient number and my date of birth.

"You are all set. Let me show you to your room. This is the room you will wait in before the surgery and the room you will come back to after the procedure." The woman said as we walked down the hallway. "Just to confirm you have not eaten or drank anything since 12:00 a.m. this morning?"

"No, I mean no, I have not eaten or drank anything," I reply, having my early morning brain fog show a little more than I meant it to.

"Great, well, this is your room. Room one. Your nurse will be in shortly to take your vitals and history. In the meantime, if you don't mind getting changed into this gown, socks, and hairnet, that would be fantastic."

"Sounds good, thank you!"

"Best of luck." The woman said, turning to leave my room.

I quickly get changed, putting my comfortable sweatshirt, leggings, and socks in my marathon bag, and changing them out for a gown, hair net, and grippy socks. Goosebumps form on my arms as I try to get comfortable in what I can assume is an infusion chair.

Like always, my mother starts joking around, trying to take my mind off of what is soon to happen. Once she runs out of things to joke about, reality hits me once more. Not that I have time to worry about it, as my phone buzzes in my hand. I open it to see that it's a text from my best friend, Nellie.

Hey, I don't know if you will see this before your surgery but Al and I are thinking of you, we love you so much! Text me once you are out!

Attached to that message is a picture of her, my friend Allie, and me from the previous night. We met up at Allie's house for what we were calling 'Ruth's final supper'. It was fun. We ate, danced, and joked. The best part was we all are on summer vacation and both of them woke up at 6:30 to wish me good luck. *I love my friends.* Then another woman walked in. "Hi, I'm Carla. I will be your surgical nurse today. Can you please tell me your full name and date of birth?"

"Ruth Louise Bilbruck, and 07/27/2007."

"Amazing, and you are here today for an endoscopy."

"Yep."

"K, I'm going to take your vitals; and then your anesthesiologist is going to come in and get an IV in you, and then you will be set for a 7:00 a.m. procedure."

"Amazing, thank you," I responded.

We started off with my height and weight, then my blood pressure, and blood, for what I am guessing is a pregnancy test, then my pulse and heart rate.

Once that was done, my anesthesiologist came in. "Hi, Ruth."

She's tall, with beautiful, long, black hair and dark brown eyes. She looks very young, which shocks me as she is the anesthesiologist.

"My name is Dr. Begum and I will be your anaesthesiologist today." I tip my head to say hi.

"Hi."

"Is this your first time going under general?" Dr. Begum asks, grabbing a kit from the cabinet behind me.

"Yes," I reply, turning to see what the kit has in it.

"Well, for our teens, we put in the IV before we put you under, so the side effects of the anesthesia are limited. Can I please have the hand you want the IV in?"

I gave her my left as I am right-handed, and I am hoping to do some school prep after this.

"Great, now this is a needle, but it is just going to poke you and then it will leave this super cool port in you so we can put your medication in during your surgery."

I HATE it when doctors talk to me like I'm four. I understand that I am treated at a children's hospital. I am on the older end of the spectrum, but I know it says in my chart that I want to be a neurosurgeon when I grow up. I have seen hundreds of IVs placed on the internet during my personal training. I know what is going to happen. I smile and nod my head instead of saying any of that.

"So, this is going to hurt. We recommend you look at your mom so you don't flinch."

"I will be ok, thank you though. I can watch my own blood get drawn. Needles don't really scare me anymore." I said, looking at my mom, who is looking anywhere but my hand. She HATES needles.

"Ok, sounds good to me. Would you like me to count or just put it in?"

"Either works for me," I respond, looking at my left hand as she tries to find a vein.

Even though I talk a lot, I truly don't like needles. I mean, I can watch them. I am better than I was when I was younger;

not crying and running away from the nurse is a very small improvement. My stomach still starts to turn when I realize what is coming.

"One, Two, Three."

As the needle pushes through my skin I gasp. That *hurts a lot more than getting your blood drawn.* For a second, I thought it entered my center metacarpal bone. My hand was not growing in size, so I assumed not. The pain went away quickly after the puncture. She flushes it with saline. I can feel the cold liquid flooding down my hand. I'm scared for a minute that the IV has been removed and its blood running down my hand. My fear is quickly depleted when I notice that it's still in place. My mother is called out of the room to finish up some paperwork. I see it as my chance to start my second plan of the day.

"Do you mind passing me my bag?" I ask Dr. Begum.

"Sure."

As she gets it for me, I start on the speech I had planned. "So, I read on the Seattle Children's website that patients can ask to have something placed under their pillow while they are having a procedure and I know I am a little over the age, but I would really appreciate it." I pull out my rag of a pink blanket out of my bag. "Also, if my mom could not find out that I brought this, that would be amazing. It will just make her nervous." I said, passing her the blanket.

"Of course. I will have a nurse slip it into your bag when your mom is signing your discharge papers."

"Thank you so much!"

She leaves right as my mom enters the room.

"So, what did you and her talk about?" My mom asks.

"Just the usual, any drug use, or is there any chance you're pregnant?" I reply by putting my bag back on the chair next to my mom.

"And I am almost positive that I know the answer, and both are 'no'?"

"Yes mom, both are 'no'. When would I have time for that, anyway? If I'm not with you, I'm at school, and I would not trust the kids there to not have some disease, and the boys at my school are disgusting."

"K, I'm just checking."

"I know, and I love you for it. You just need to know I am not going to cause myself any more health issues than I already have." I reach out for my mom's hand, and I rub it.

Carla comes back in shortly after that. "It looks like the OR is ready for you. We're going to put you in a wheelchair and then take you down. I'll give you a minute, and then when you are ready, feel free to open the door and one of our OR nurses will come and get you. Good luck!"

"Thank you," I replied, turning toward my mom. She has tears in her eyes, and I start to feel sick. "Mom, I'm going to be ok. After this, we're going to go to Funko, right?"

"Yep, sweety," my mom said slowly as if she is trying not to fall apart.

"I think I'm going to look for the new Loki Funkos."

"Whatever you want, you get two." I stare at her for a minute, trying to remember every inch of her face as it might be the last time I saw her.

"Mom, I love you so much."

Now I'm the one trying to hold back tears. Though endoscopies are low risk, you never know what will happen.

"Thank you for being my hero."

My mom gets up and embraces me in a hug. "I love you too, Ruthbear. You are one of my greatest achievements. I love you!"

I hug her back, not even caring that the pressure she is putting on my body is hurting my nerves. I would risk my life for my mom. It's unexplainably hard to think this could be the last time I would see her, hold her, hear 'I love you' from her. Then it was over. She gets up and nods at me. I nod back, and she opens the door. The OR nurse, Shannon, came in and got me situated in the wheelchair.

As I was being rolled out, I said, "Thank you, Mom, I love you."

And though I didn't hear it, I know she said, "I love you, too, honey."

present Day

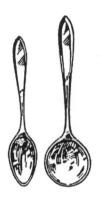

The questions and sympathy decay my brain like time does to trash as I continue my day at the pain clinic. When I see Dr. McMelson, she does a thorough physical examination. She has all of my vitals retaken, even though I had already done it today, and checks every inch of my body for any marks or abrasions. She explains that my body is amplifying my pain like a speaker does to music. She explains this by taking a wooden stick and pressing it into my back. It feels like a knife going into my back, even though it is dull. She takes her finger and does the same thing. I cannot feel the difference between her fingers and the stick. Both feel like a hot poker; like I am a fire on a cold night, and someone is using a poker to rearrange my wood. I start to feel sick. Stomach pain and nausea are a part of this mystery I call my life. I ask Dr. McMelson for a vomit bag.

"Yes, of course," she said, reaching for one. I take it and nod my thanks.

"So, what can we do?" my mother asks, playing with her bracelet like she does every time she gets nervous.

"I will meet with the rest of the team, and we will figure something out. Then, at your last meeting of the day, Dr. Wilson will tell you the treatment plan and what to look forward to in the future."

"Thank you," I said, trying to relax my breathing as my Biofeedback therapist, George, has taught me. She leaves, and five minutes later I hear two knocks on the door, and respond by saying come in. Dr. Wilson walks in and starts by asking my mom to leave the room. Which isn't unordinary. He's a pain psychologist. I'm over thirteen. My mental health information is private only to me.

He starts off by reintroducing himself, saying, "So we have already met, but it was early when we did. So let me reintroduce myself. I am Dr. Wilson. My pronouns are he/him, and I will be your pain psychologist. Now, what does that mean for you? Well, I'm going to help you deal with the emotions and feelings you are having as a person with chronic pain because there aren't a lot of kids who you know that will understand this. Now, before we start, I want to remind you that because you're over thirteen, I can't tell your mom anything we talk about in these rooms without your permission. Now that's out of the way. Tell me how you're feeling today."

"My pain is at level six," I responded.

"Not your pain level. How are you mentally and emotionally feeling?"

Honestly, I didn't know how to respond because I haven't been doing so well. I feared being moved to inpatient treatment, so I kept that part to myself.

"I've been good."

"Your life is just good? It's almost like you don't have chronic pain?"

"I do, but I'm good, happy."

"Ok, have you ever been depressed?"

"Yeah, a couple years ago, but I'm better now, really," I respond by trying to smile so he believes me.

He pulls out a sheet of paper and a pencil and asks me to write out my family tree. I am shocked but comply. *The sooner I make this stupid tree, the sooner I get out of here.* As I draw and write down the names of my family, I see him going through my medical history in his glasses' reflection. It looks like a novel. When I finish, I give him back the clipboard.

"So, you live with your mom and sister?"

"Yes."

"And who's Bruce?"

"That's my mom's boyfriend. He's around a lot, so I didn't know where to put him," I respond, rubbing my arm up and down with my hand.

"And John, his name is off to the side?" Dr. Wilson asked, pointing to it.

"That's my dad. I haven't talked to him in a little while, since he left my family for his mistress," I respond quietly, hoping that I won't have to answer anymore about him.

My father and I don't talk anymore, so there isn't a reason to continue talking about him. He left. That's life.

"I'm sorry about that, Ruth, and how long ago was that?"

"About a half-a-year ago, but I don't care anymore. I start high school next year. I can't continue to be mad that my dad never loved me like TV said he would," I said, chuckling, but then realizing that was probably not the right thing to say.

There continued to be more of that, asking about my feelings and what's going on in my life just for me to say the bare minimum. I have seen a therapist before, and they are all the same. Except my current therapist, Morgan, who just gets me. She's the type of therapist that lets me talk about whatever I want, even if that's sometimes a TV show or movie I watched. She also has tons of toys and fidgets in her office and snacks that I can eat while there. I hated the idea of therapy, but now I feel weird if I do not see her at least once a week. It took me a long time to get there with her, so the fact that Dr. Wilson just wants me to open up about my deepest battles after meeting him less than an hour ago makes me chuckle.

"Well, that is all I need. It was nice to meet you, Ruth, and I will see you later." Dr. Wilson stands up, shakes my hand, and leaves; leaves the room, and leaves me with thousands of questions.

seven months prior

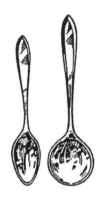

To Do List For School:

-Talk to teachers about Chronic Illness

-Get Note to Front office, nurse, and gym teacher

-Email Counselor about 504 plan

I look at my to-do list for the first day of school. Man, it would be amazing if my only thing was to have fun and pick a good locker. Of course, there's medical things to do. It feels like there always is. I sent a text to my friends Nellie, Alexa, Asher, Nicole, and Emma.

Meet at the table on the second level for lunch today, I can't wait to hear about all of your first days!!!

As I send it, the bell rings for the first period. After the beginning of the school year ice breakers, we are given a break to chat with some of our classmates. I use this time to talk to my English teacher, Mrs. Kenny.

"Mrs. Kenny, do you think we can talk outside for a minute?" I ask in my sweetest voice.

"Yes, of course." She gets up from her desk.

My palms start to sweat, and my knees get weak. *I should make business cards that are like, 'Hi, I have numerous chronic illnesses, thanks for understanding. It would make this so much easier.'*

"What's up?" She asks, as she closes the door.

"So, I just wanted to let you know that I have a chronic illness called AMPS or Amplified Musculoskeletal Pain Syndrome, which means that my body is in pain twenty-four-seven. I also have undiagnosed GI issues and chronic fatigue disorder. And for all of this, I am treated at Seattle Children's. Now I am not telling you this as an excuse. I have just learned that telling my teachers sooner rather than later is actually super helpful. And I am a hard-working student. I have great grades and I am really excited to take your course this year. And I have a doctor's note if you want to see it, but it is also in my 504 plan." I take a breath for the first time since starting to speak.

"Wow, I am sorry you have to deal with this. Is there anything I can do to best support you in my class?" Mrs. Kenny asks.

These are the good responses. Not the teachers who think they know what you're going through or try to fix you. She just wants to best support me.

"Sometimes I might have to turn in things later than usual because I am having a flare-up or my appointments are keeping me from doing it, but I am very good at communicating these things before the due date. The main thing is I have some treatments I have to do while I am in class. Like if my stomach hurts, I have a portable cordless heating pad, or if I'm nauseous, I have medication for that. So, nothing on your side, just being aware that this is something I struggle with." I reply, trying to smile, even though having these conversations makes me feel like a part of my soul is dying.

"Thank you for telling me. I am very excited for this school year and to have you in my class." She said, opening the door.

One down, five more to go.

present Day

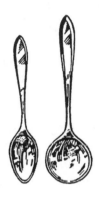

I am at the appointment I had been longing for and dreading at the same time. I will finally receive a diagnosis, a reason for my suffering, light at the end of the tunnel. As I glanced at my mom, I saw a flicker of fear in her eyes. Though I was the only one that could tell because everyone else would think it was an eyelash. She worried that we spent a whole day for nothing and that she put her daughter through more poking and prodding to just be told there is nothing they could do.

I heard two knocks on the door, and for the final time that day I weakly called out, "Come in."

Dr. Wilson greeted us and thanked us for the billionth time that day for coming down on such short notice. He was wearing the same half zip sweater he was wearing that morning and continued to wear his 'I love my dog' pin. He had two papers in his hands. One thing I have learned is that papers are usually bad. From transfer notes to screening information, the papers never leave me with a smile on my face. Not being able to read Dr. Wilson's facial expressions because of the mask due to the pandemic made the conversation long and strenuous. Dr. Wilson showed me the first paper.

"So as a future neurosurgeon like yourself, I'm going to explain this in a way you will understand. Your body's nerves are messed up. There is an abnormal short circuit in the spinal cord. The normal pain signal not only travels up to the brain but also goes to the neurovascular nerves that control blood flow through the blood vessels. These nerves cause the blood vessels to become smaller. This constriction restricts blood flow and oxygen to muscles and bone and leads to an increase in waste products, such as lactic acid. It is this lack of oxygen and acid build-up that causes pain. Does that make sense?" Dr. Wilson said, finally taking a breath and turning toward me.

And for some weird reason, it did.

"Yeah, actually it does," I said, standing up to stretch. I had been sitting for too long and my body was starting to hate me.

"No, no, it doesn't. Explain it to someone who has not gone to medical school or watched all of *Grey's Anatomy*." My mother said, proud of me but wanting to understand it herself.

"Ruth's nerves are misfiring in her spine and causing more pain, and because Ruth didn't get the right diagnoses for so long and her doctors were treating it wrong, it has spread and become increasingly worse."

"So, what can we do?" My mom asked, for the first time in two years, with a little bit of hope in her voice.

"It's going to be long and hard, but Ruth's strong. She's going to make it through this." He said, going on to talk about a five-stage plan to even get me back to living a semi-normal life. Though a semi-normal life is the bare minimum that I need.

When you get a diagnosis, it rocks your world. Your thoughts on life change.

As I exited the hospital, the cold air hit my face. The world seems to slow down as I walk to my car. I notice the other patients walking into the hospital, clinging to their parents. I notice the signs on the flag poles saying, "Seattle Children's is the home of hope," and I start to feel sick. To me, this diagnosis was not a sign of hope but a life sentence. I saw it as another way the universe was trying to get me hopeful and then was going to kick my knees. The fact that the pain was going to continue to spread and there was no way to stop it left me with a pit in my stomach. I get into my car and rip off my purple hospital band. I tore the band up like the doctors did to my hope and then I went numb. Of course, not physically as exhausting pain continues throughout my body. But my soul felt numb. Like every time I got my hopes up, and I was proven wrong, I lost a piece of myself. I started identifying as my chronic illness. Living for my treatments instead of doing my treatments so I could live. I lost myself in the process.

FOUR MONTHS PRIOR

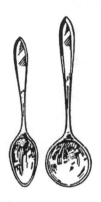

When I walk into Seattle Children's Northern. I quickly get checked in and run to the bathroom to get changed. I'm the only one in the bathroom, which is completely normal. I take the biggest stall to get changed in. I came straight from school, so I am in my school clothes (A sweater with a pair of slacks and black shoes) and I get changed into my old band t-shirt, black leggings, and Adidas sneakers. I tie up my shoes, thinking about the reason I am wearing Adidas. My old soccer coach had a huge thing for Adidas. I started buying them exclusively. I shove my clothes in my bag, not caring they will probably wrinkle and exit the stall. I deep wash my hands, clean from my elbow to the tip of my fingers. *I have finals coming up. I do not have time to be sick.* When I exit the bathroom, I stop by the vending machine and pick up a protein bar. Even though I would usually prefer a fresher choice, it was the best thing in it. I had not eaten since breakfast because I ended up working through my lunch. I didn't want to risk passing out again. As I sit down, I am met by the annoying pity glances from the parents sitting with their children. It's funny to me that they seem to care that I am here alone, while I don't. I prefer coming to my appointments alone. When I do, the doctors talk to me not my mother. I unwrap the protein bar and take a bite. It's not great, kind of like chalk. I alternate between a bite from the bar and a drink of water. I am trying to force the bar down when I look up to see a teen about my age come in alone. As a longtime resident of this waiting room, I know almost all chronic patients who come alone, but somehow, I don't know this one. They check in; I figure out how I am going to start a conversation. I mean, if I have to wait, it would be nice to have someone to talk to. They walk over and sit two chairs away from me on the same wall. I notice that they are fidgeting with their hospital band. In my years of studying, I know that means they are probably newer, or even their first time. So, I work up the courage and use the only line I know in my book,

"Is this your first time?" I ask.

"Yeah, how could you tell?" The patient asked, turning to face me.

"Two things, one, you are fidgeting with your hospital band, and two, you have not memorized the intake questions. You are still thinking about the answers." I reply, reaching out my hand so she can shake it. "My name is Ruth, and I use she/her pronouns."

"Lizzie and I use she/they pronouns." They replied, shaking my hand.

"So, I have to ask, what are you here for?" Hoping this is not too personal.

"I have chronic depression disorder and I am here for Biofeedback therapy. And you?"

"Chronic pain, and today I am here for physical therapy, but tomorrow I am here for Biofeedback, and the next day I am here for a social worker meeting," I said. "Are you seeing George?"

"Yeah, he seems nice from the videos I watch about Biofeedback, but I'm still kind of worried," Lizzie replied.

"I can tell you from personal experience that he is the sweetest, most caring person ever. And he has a really good sense of humor." I said, trying to comfort her, noticing George walk out of the hallway behind us.

"Elizebeth," he calls out.

"That's me, but I go as Lizzie." They correct him as they stand up. "It was really nice to talk to you, Ruth. Thank you."

I nod back, "Have fun," waving at George, who nods back at me.

present day

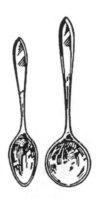

As I walk into Seattle Children's Northern Clinic, I pause for a minute. I see the patients and parents waiting in the waiting area; I see the holiday decorations behind the front desk, and I notice the other receptionist chatting about something. I notice the safe, even home-like feeling I get when I walk through the sliding doors. A feeling I had never noticed before. I walk to the front desk. Chase motions for me to come to his stall. Walking there, I notice how I started looking at Chase the same way I do to my friends at school. Knowing that, if need be, they will be there for me.

"The amazing Ruth Bilbruck!" I said, as I reached his stall. Doing some weird dramatic stance like I was the queen of the world.

"Hey Ruth," Chase said, rolling his eyes at my dramatic personality. "How did that test go? The one you were worried about last time."

"Good, I got a four on it so that was cool," I said, reaching for the purple hospital band that Chase is handing me. "Thanks."

"Have fun with Mark!" Chase said, smiling at me.

I turned around and gave him the swag boy pose and walked to the waiting room. It has been two weeks since my diagnosis, and I have finally started to feel like myself again. I'm not a chronic pain patient; I'm a patient with chronic pain. I realized I wasn't and did not need to become my chronic illness. I didn't have to be the sick girl. I could continue to be Ruth even though I had to go to treatments three times a week and my closest friends are now my treatment nurse, Dr. Wilson, and Mark. I am still a teen and can live a teen-ish life. It's my life and I get to choose what I want to do with it. I thought about this as I sat in the waiting room. I turned as I heard someone walking down the hall behind me.

"Ruth, you ready?" Mark said, turning to head back down the hall.

"Yeah, give me a sec," I said, collecting my things and walking toward him.

"How have you been?" He asked.

"Fine," I said. "You?"

"I've been good, busy but good." He said this as we entered the PT gym.

I put my things down and jumped on the treadmill.

"What are you thinking about? You're making your weird thinking face." He said, starting the treadmill.

"Have you ever noticed that you never know you have an ability until you lose it?" I said, looking at him. "Mine was the ability to walk pain-free."

WORKS CITED

Miserandino. Christine. "The Spoon Theory". But You Don't Look Sick, 2003,

https://butyoudontlooksick.com/category/the-spoon-theory/

ABOUT RILEY BOERGER

I want to start off by thanking you for reading my book. As a 15 year old in a small town in Washington, this is a dream I never thought I could reach. Everything I wrote about is based on personal experiences. Writing this book was very therapeutic. A little about me: I use pronouns she/her, I will be in 10th grade this upcoming school year (meaning that I will have a published book before my high school diploma), and I want to be a neurosurgeon when I am older. I always believe that my age does not stop me from reaching the stars. I am so excited to share this with you. Remember your past does not define you.

Connect with me:

Instagram- riley_boerger

TikTok- Chronically_riley

Email- Rileyboerget@icloud.com

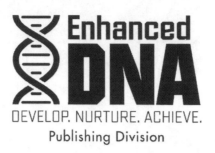

Enhanced DNA
DEVELOP. NURTURE. ACHIEVE.
Publishing Division

Made in the USA
Las Vegas, NV
05 September 2022

54730169R00050